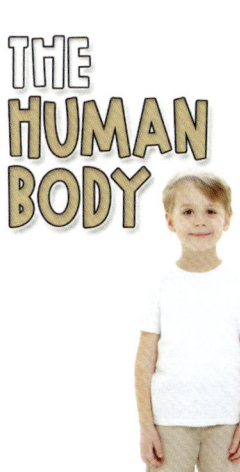

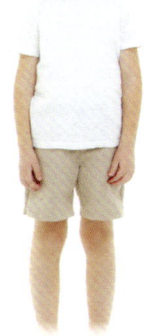

Written By: Anna DiGilio

All rights reserved. No part of this publication may be reproduced, distributed, or transmitted in any form or by any means, including photocopying, recording, or other electronic or mechanical methods, without the prior written permission of the publisher, except in the case of brief quotations embodied in critical reviews and certain other noncommercial uses permitted by copyright law.

For permission requests, write to the publisher:
Laprea Publishing
info@lapreapublishing.com

Website: www.GuidedReaders.com

ISBN: 978-1-64579-991-7

© 2020 Anna DiGilio

Photo Credits:
Cover, Title Page: Shutterstock; Sergei Kolesnikov. 3: Shutterstock; MarShot. 4: Shutterstock; Karelnoppe. 5 (edited), 6 (edited), 7 (top), 7 (center; edited), 8 (edited), 9 (edited), 10 (edited): Shutterstock; Vecton. 11 (edited): Shutterstock; Medicalstocks. 12 (edited): Shutterstock; Karelnoppe. 13 (top): Shutterstock; Hung Chung Chih. 13 (center): Shutterstock; New Africa. 13 (bottom): Shutterstock; Szefei.

TABLE OF CONTENTS

Your Body .... Page 4

Bones .... Page 5

Muscles .... Page 6

Lungs .... Page 7

Heart .... Page 8

Brain .... Page 9

Stomach .... Page 10

Kidneys .... Page 11

Other Body Parts .... Page 12

Help Your Body .... Page 13

Glossary .... Page 14

Your Body

Your body has many parts. They do many jobs. They work as a team. They keep you alive and well.

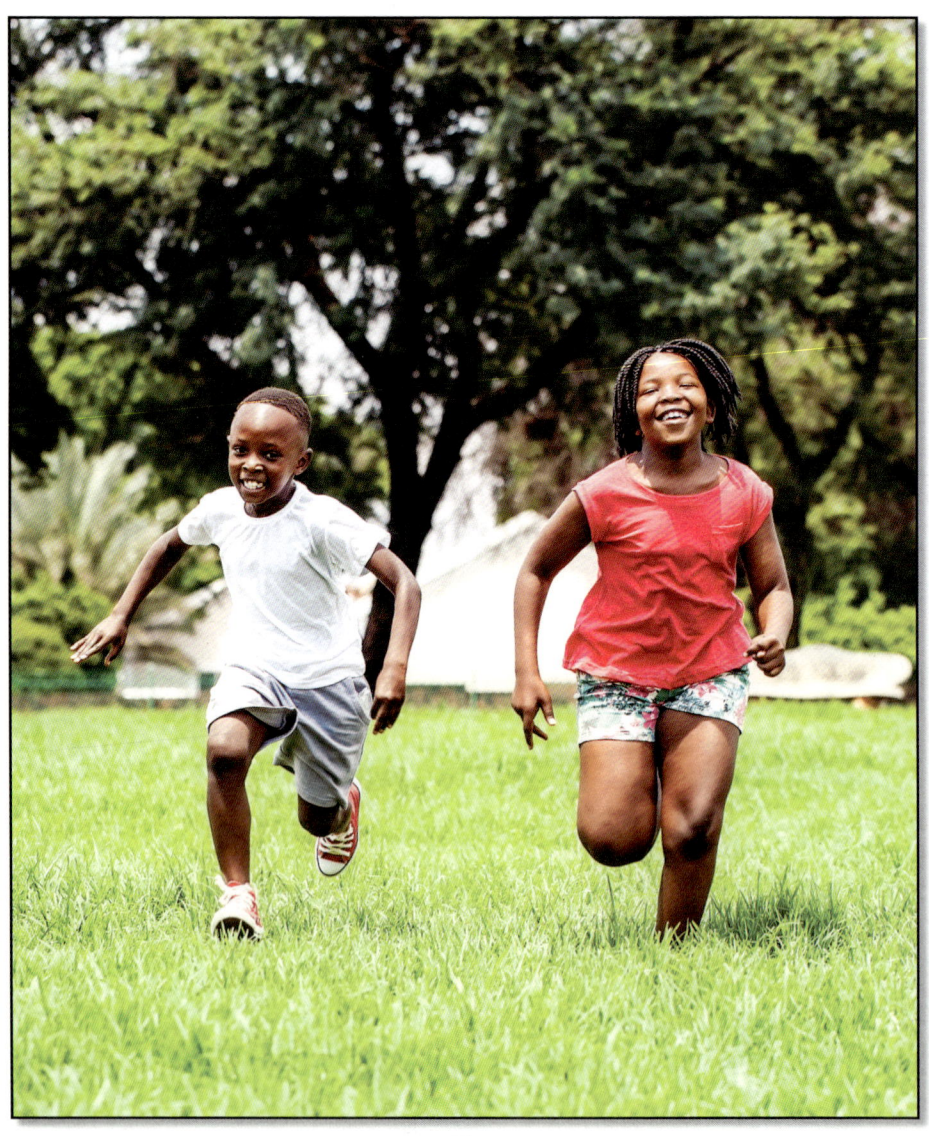

Bones

These body parts are hard. They hold up your body. They let you move. They have many shapes.

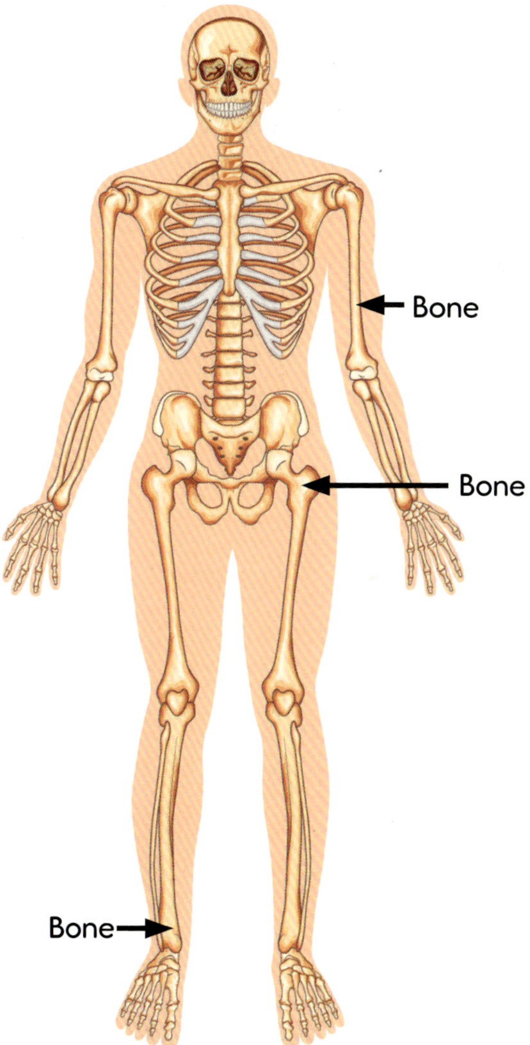

← Bone

← Bone

Bone →

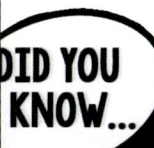

DID YOU KNOW...

Bones are alive! Bones grow longer. They also grow and heal if they break.

Muscles

These body parts help you move. They help you walk. They help you eat. They help you do many things!

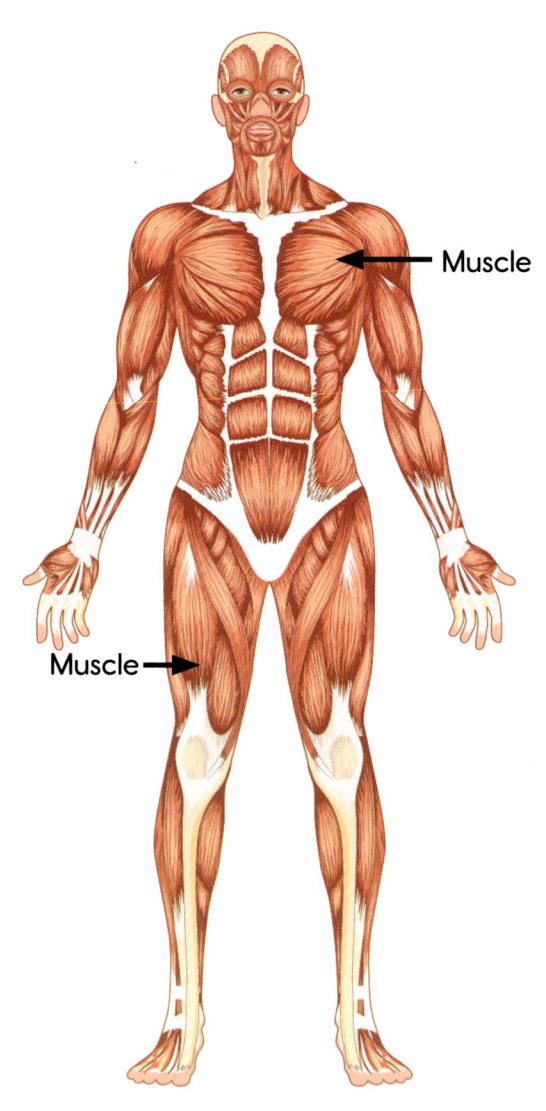

Lungs

These body parts help you take in air. <u>Breathe</u> in. Breathe out. Breathe deep. Breathe out.

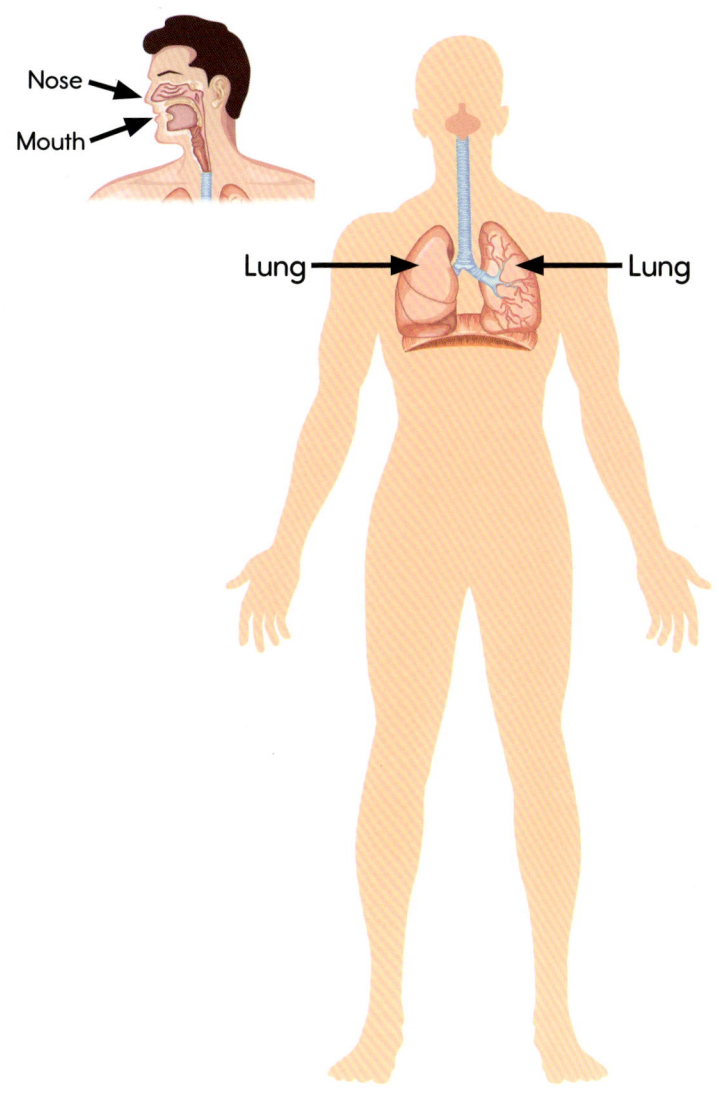

Heart

This body part moves <u>blood</u>. Blood goes to all body parts. Blood keeps you alive. Thank you, blood!

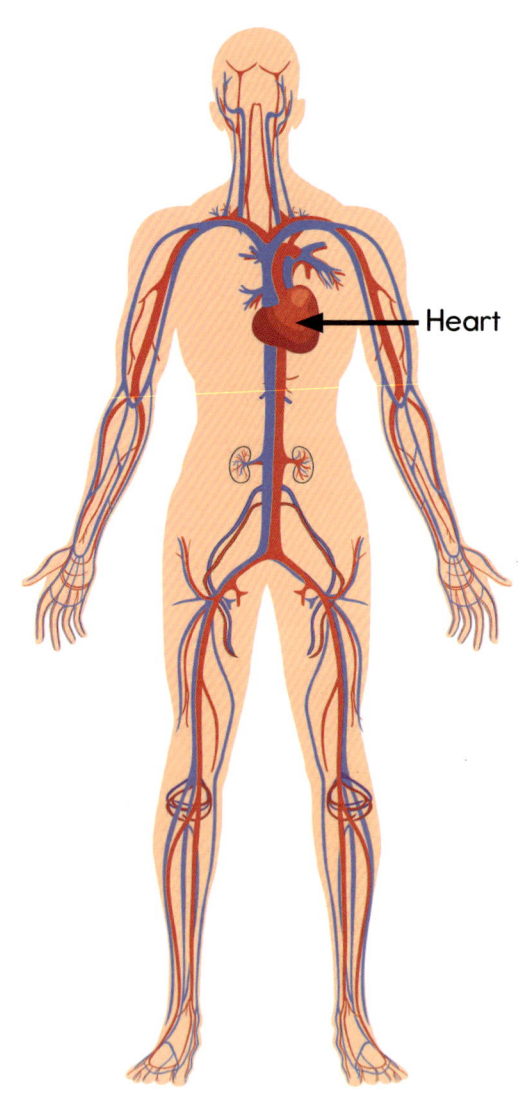
Heart

Brain

This body part helps you think. It helps you feel. It helps you move, too.

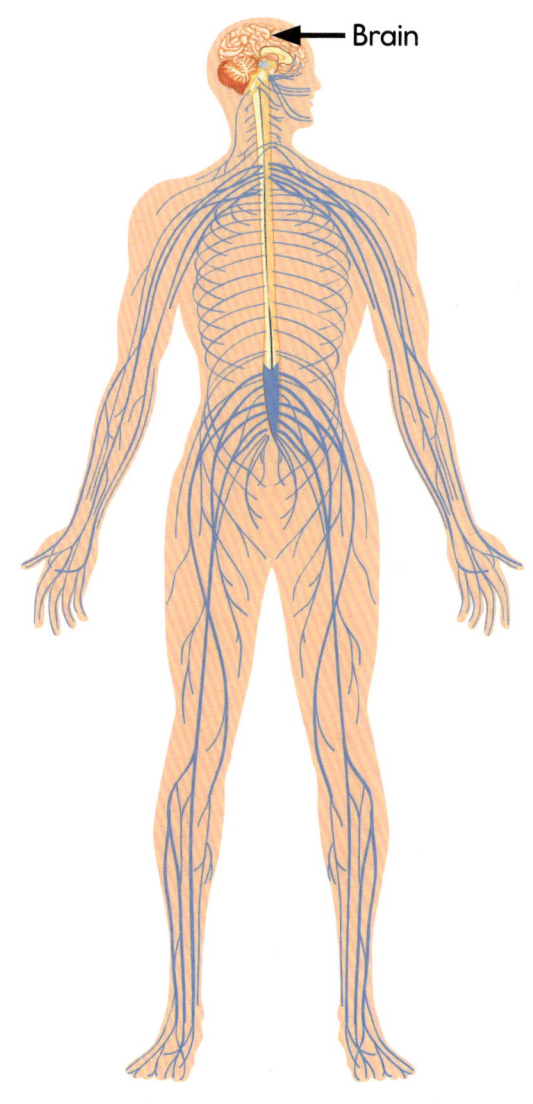

Stomach

You eat food. Food helps your body do work. This body part helps your body use food. It breaks food into small pieces. Other body parts help, too!

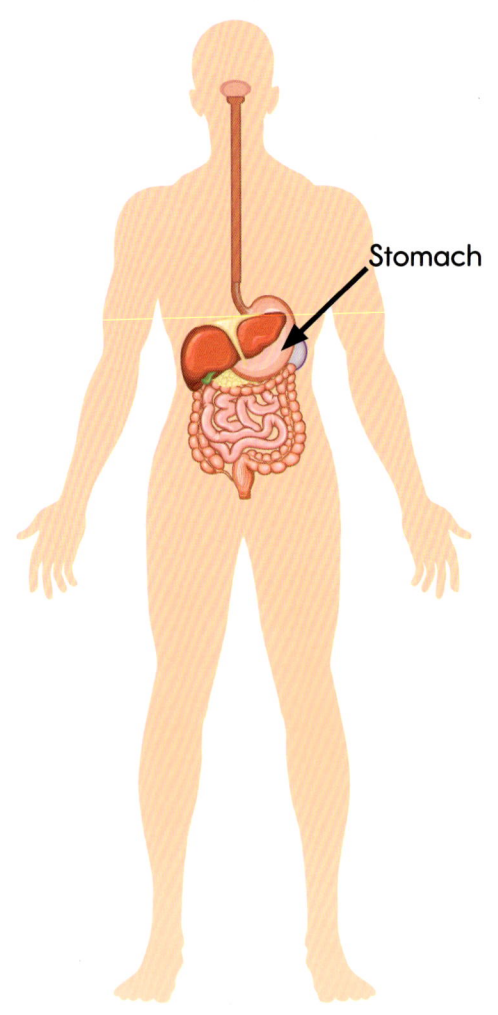

Kidneys

Blood goes through these body parts. They make your blood <u>clean</u>. They take out dirt. They mix it with water. It goes to another part. Then it leaves your body.

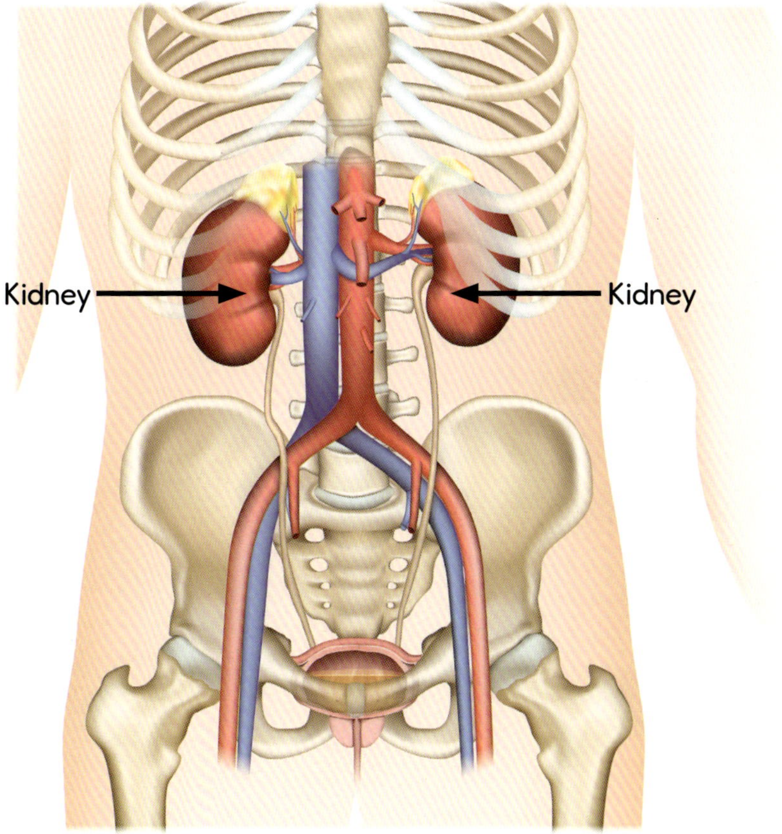

Kidney ⟶   ⟵ Kidney

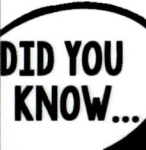

DID YOU KNOW... You have two kidneys. But you only need one. Some people lose a kidney. The other one grows bigger!

Other Body Parts

You have other body parts, too. Some help you grow. Some help you stay well.

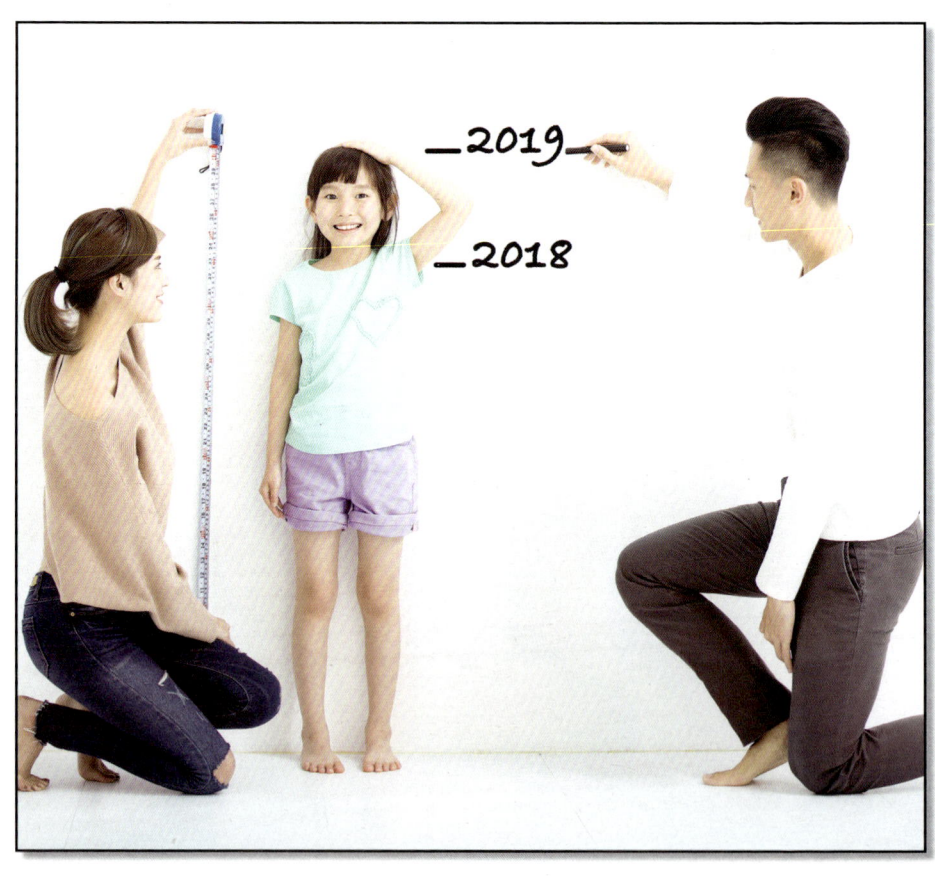

Help Your Body

Your body has many jobs. It keeps you well. You can help.
- Get enough sleep.
- Do not sit too much. Move!
- Eat food that is good for you.

Take care of your body!

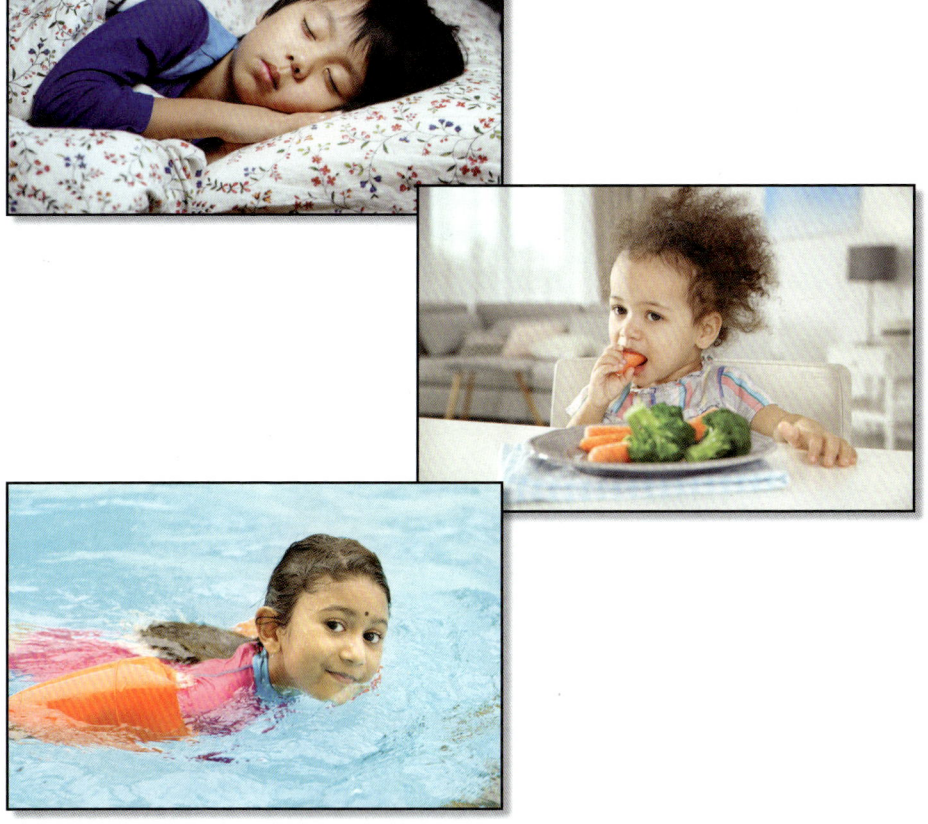

GLOSSARY

<u>blood</u>
the red liquid inside the body of a person or other animal

<u>breathe</u>
to take in and let out air through the nose and mouth

<u>clean</u>
not dirty